Sex

for

BUSY PEOPLE

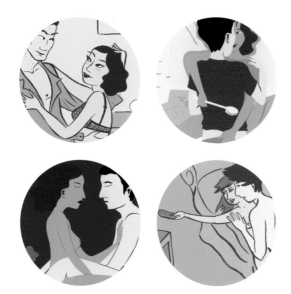

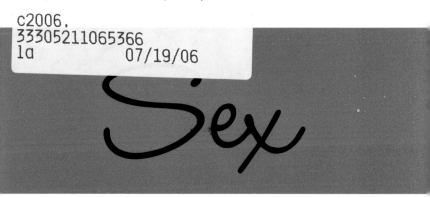

Sex

for

BUSY PEOPLE

by Emily Dubberley

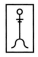

A FIRESIDE BOOK
PUBLISHED BY SIMON & SCHUSTER
NEW YORK LONDON TORONTO SYDNEY

FIRESIDE
Rockefeller Center
1230 Avenue of the Americas
New York, NY 10020

FIRESIDE and colophon are registered trademarks
of Simon & Schuster, Inc.

Conceived and produced by
Elwin Street Limited
79 St John Street
London EC1M 4NR
www.elwinstreet.com

For information regarding special discounts for bulk
purchases, please contact Simon & Schuster Special
Sales at 1-800-456-6798 or business@simonandschuster.com.

Designed by Kelly Blair
Illustrated by Leela Corman
With thanks to Sam Hiyate and Kim Hartness for editorial help

Manufactured in Singapore

10 9 8 7 6 5 4 3 2 1

Library of Congress Cataloging-in-Publication data is available

ISBN-13: 978-0-7432-8468-4
ISBN-10:   0-7432-8468-2

Contents

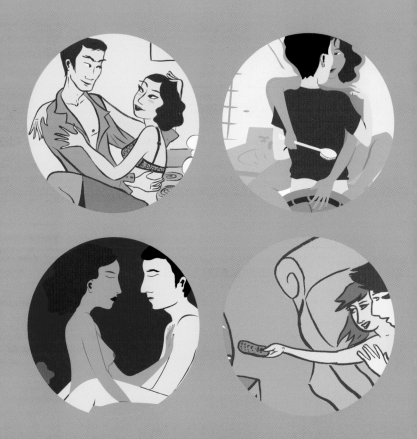

Introduction

Forget Tantric sex, welcome to frantic sex. Fast, furious fun that promises orgasms in less time than it takes to make coffee. This is turbo-charged passion, perfect for those times when you want great sex and you want it now! Quality quickies, where you tear at each other's clothes, wreck the bed, and still make it back downstairs by the end of the commercial break.

Good quickies are about delirious, delicious sex that's just as good (and sometimes better!) as the kind you'd have in your comfortable bed with time for fabulous foreplay. There's no right time or place for a quickie. If you really need it, want it, or are simply thinking about it, you'll find a way to communicate your sense of urgency. The kitchen table or the garden shed will do.

If you've ever wanted to learn how to deliver the perfect blow job in under 10 minutes, give yourself an orgasm in less than five, or fit amazing, three-position lovemaking into your lunch hour, you've come to the right place. We've stripped sex down to its bare essentials, giving you all the tips you've ever needed to become famous for your 15-minute nookie. We'll tell you the naughtiest locations and best positions to grab a quick one. We'll tell you the pleasure points on your body that will turn you from Off to On within seconds. And we'll even tell you the secret to having amazing sex at a party where you can come before anyone realizes you've gone.

For people who are juggling two busy schedules, who want to inject instant intensity back into their bedroom, or for those who just crave the rush of the rush, this is the only book you'll ever need.

Fast love starts right now.

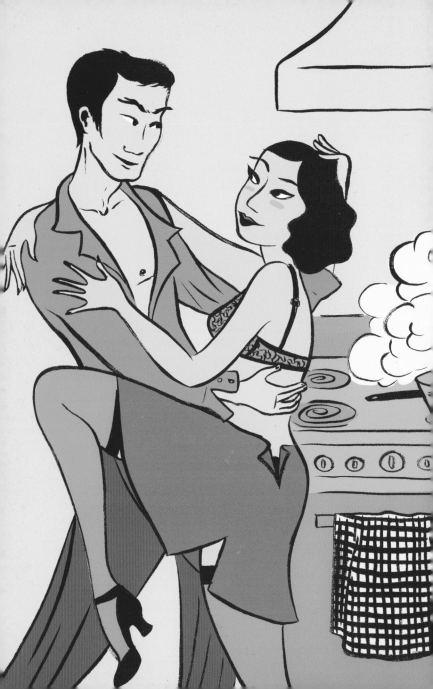

5 Minutes

The in-laws are coming over for brunch, the kids are tidying up their rooms and, since you're making hard-boiled eggs, you consider for a moment how nice it is when your lover is hard and you're boiling over with desire. Now is the time to act on it! These scenarios are perfect for those moments when you're almost out of time, and yet you'd rather not eat until you and your lover are satiated first.

There She Blows

His cock can go from a standing start to spurting happily in less time than it takes him to brush his teeth. Which is fabulous for oral sex. He gets instant pleasure; you don't get lockjaw.

Kneel before him, place your palms either side of his flaccid member, and roll it between them. Think "girl guide trying to start a fire" (because that's what you're doing).

After a minute or so, take his erect cock deep into your mouth. Use your tongue to stimulate the head. Cup his balls in your left hand, and use your right thumb to massage the underside of his head. Increase the ball-massage, slipping your hand under his balls to massage his perineum. Slide him as far back as possible into your throat, moaning in delight. Increase both speed and pressure and, once you hear his moans, you'll know you've reignited the home fires.

Kiss Me Slow

Remember those hot and steamy first-date French-kissing sessions that caused your knees to tremble and your pussy to tingle? When the kissing stops, so can the passion. So reintroduce this underrated erotic activity.

Try to squeeze a some tonsil tennis in every day by turning your goodbye kiss or your usual peck on the cheek into something gorgeously memorable. Don't you want him to leave you at least a little wet?

To turn any kiss into a knee-trembling inferno, first think "seduction." By holding this word in mind, your tongue will instinctively produce the most seductive kiss imaginable. Secondly, imagine you are giving head. Give his tongue a slow, sensuous blow job, gently sucking it, running your mouth up and down it, playing with the tip.

Explore the roof of his mouth—it is highly sensitive. If he's not a natural kisser, help him. Ask him to kiss the tip of your tongue as if it was your clit.

Warning: French kissing may not only bring back fabulous memories of your teenage years and first dates, it can become addictive and will mean completely re-doing your lipstick.

Stairway to Heaven

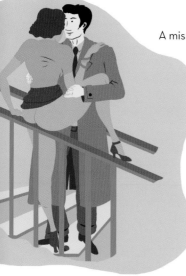

A mismatch in heights can make sex standing up tricky to pull off, but a quickie on the stairs provides the perfect height equalizer. Try this at home, or if it's a spontaneous lunchtime quickie, head to the deserted stairwell of a building with an elevator, preferably on a high floor.

Position one: If you're shorter than your man, stand a step or two up from him and place one leg over the railing so that you can both maintain motion and balance. (If he's shorter, he can stand a step or two up from you.) Tilt your pelvis so that your pussy is forward.

Position two: Present your rear and bend over slightly, inviting him to enter. You can grip onto the rail for leverage.

Dress code: Skirt for you, raincoat for him. That way, if a fitness freak decides to take the stairs, you can part and hide any evidence—other than your smiles and flushed faces, of course.

Circuit Training

Your man was created with 10 fingers. And now is the time to make use of three of them. In the same way that a three-pronged plug creates a surge of electricity when inserted into the appropriate socket, this technique is perfect—especially when time is of the essence—for sending a lightning bolt through your body.

His pre-licked or lubricated thumb should softly circle you, with his thumb focusing on your clitoral bud. His index finger should gently probe your pussy lips and environs. As the index finger starts to edge further inside you, invited by your natural wetness, his ring finger should approach the rosebud of your anus—an area with equally sensitive nerve endings. All three fingers now cover all three bases, and they should be attending to them with a strong rhythm to work their combined magic.

Since he is just using one hand, he could of course also lick, fondle, or otherwise titillate the rest of you at the same time. With intense attention on all your pleasure zones, expect a short, sharp shock when you come.

Car-nal Knowledge

Engaging in foreplay while one of you is driving is always a bad idea. But if you don't mind being a little late to your evening soirée, he might appreciate a member massage once you're parked. If it's dark outside, the location won't matter, but if it's still daylight, pull over into a quiet, out-of-the-way parking lot, or even an underground one.

Next, liberate his penis and glide it into your fist-shaped palm for a quick hand job. Bring your hand down, stroking his cock from the head to the base. When you hit the bottom, move back up. Keep the pressure firm and the rhythm steady.

For a change of pace, open your palm and swirl around the head, first in one direction, then the other, before returning to the piston-pumping action.

For a different and delicious sensation, pick up a Latex glove and combine with lube or hand cream. Although you may be late, the two of you may actually be more relaxed and less frantic when you arrive at your party. And you can always blame the sticky traffic.

Cinema Paradiso

Movie theaters have long been the standard venue for first dates or for those occasional nights off from the kids. But make your evening not so standard with a little under-cover *amour*.

Once the lights have gone down, no one will question your holding hands. Or you hand resting in his lap, fondling and teasing him. Or his hand between your legs, stroking and en-couraging you through your underwear, or sliding past it and feeling you wet and eager. If you play your cards right, and you sit at the very back, you may be able to bring each other off.

Here's a tip if you know you're going to a film beforehand: Simply skip wearing underwear.

You can find lots of fun uses for the excess ice you get in cinema soft drinks, touching it to all of your most intimate parts, before it—and your partner—melts, of course.

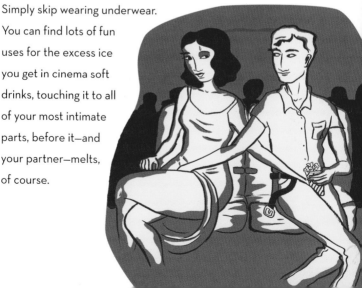

Sometimes you only see each other coming and going—in the kitchen in the morning and there again at night. So why not make it the place for a quickie? When you feel the need, you must feed the need. No-one's expecting a sit-down, five-course meal. There's not enough time to experiment with the contents of the fridge and clean the dirty dishes afterwards. This is more of a super-fast Italian sex-romp, bend-over-the-kitchen-table job.

You might want to wear sexy stockings or garters to initiate this one. And hike up your skirt to show that you are going *sans* panties.

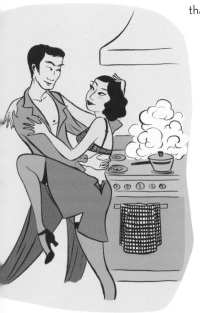

Add one firm, ripe penis and 30 hard thrusts till you are piping hot. Or, if your kitchen possesses a stepping stool as well as a free-standing washing machine, set the cycle to spin, climb onboard, spread your legs, give your man a come-hither look, and enjoy the ride.

The Pearl Necklace

This is really a treat for him, since he craves variety but doesn't always have time for an elaborate session. Massaging his cock between your breasts until he shoots and scores on your neck should ensure undying love, if not enduring memories.

Kneel in front of him while he leans over you. Essentially, you want to bun his hotdog with your breasts. If you have large breasts, use both hands to push them together to create friction as his cock slides between them. If your breasts are smaller, use one hand to cup them together and the other to navigate his cock through your valley of pleasure.

This works best post-workout, as you'll both be well-oiled with perspiration. And there will be towels nearby to mop up the pearls.

Commercial Breakdown

It's your favorite TV show and since you're not a desperate housewife, you know how to keep the horny devil on the sofa happy.

First, tell him to remove all clothes from the waist down and stay on his side of the sofa. You strip from the waist down too—easy to do without missing a moment of plot entanglement.

Then, as soon as the first ad rolls, swing into action. Lie him down and move yourself on top of him so that your clit is right in front of his lips. Your mouth, meanwhile, is hovering above his cock. You have about three and a half minutes for this 69—just the right amount of time to avoid straining your neck. Return to your sitting pose as soon as the show starts, no matter how carried away you become. After all, there'll be another break in eight minutes, when you can resume your 69. If you time it right, your climactic moment will be simultaneous with the show's— and of course, his.

Going Down

Going down in an elevator is an opportunity for him to go down, too. Glass elevators are a bad idea, unless you want an extra thrill. But during off-peak hours, an elevator that can be suspended between floors is begging for action.

If you've planned this, you will already have removed your underwear, or you are wearing a thong, which can be easily pushed aside. Don't be shy about issuing specific instructions. Suggest that he alternate his tongue between broad and pointy strokes. He should flatten the tip of his tongue for the broad stroke and narrow the tip into a point for the pointy stroke. Encourage him to use his whole face, to bury himself in your pussy. He should also insert two fingers in your pussy while licking your clit. Gentle suction is always a nice variation. Moan for encouragement.

Once you're finished and at the lobby, you might want to get on your knees and tell your man that now he's going up.

Out to Pasture

Use your five minutes of intimacy to prolong your anticipation of the next intimate encounter. Studies have shown that after 21 minutes or longer of physical foreplay, over 92 percent of women will orgasm during the resulting lovemaking session. Why not divide up those 21 minutes over the course of the day?

In the morning, help your partner dress, and touch them intimately. Over the day, find an excuse to do any of the following: kissing, talking, touching, stroking, caressing, holding, massages, back rubs, foot rubs, tickling, pinching, nibbling, hugging, licking, fondling, dancing, talking sexy.

The important thing to remember is to take your time. Be attentive and don't rush. There is no such thing as spending too much time on grazing, especially if you'll both be running off again on errands. There are no rules. Grazing encourages you to be creative in constant touching and building anticipation, so that when you do finally get naked with your partner at the end of the day, your urgent need will become a gushing release.

A Little Night Music

Guys, you should never feel threatened by introducing a vibrator into your play, especially if it's one of those nights when you're exhausted and your gorgeous lover is jumping you. There are three basic types: clitoral, G-Spot, and combination ones. But never surprise your lover with a sex toy.

To learn how she likes it best, ask your partner if you can watch them use their own vibrator. If that's fine, then ask if you can help her use it. She can put her hands over yours, so she can show you how she likes it.

Once you've gone past the initiation stage you should think of the vibrator as an addition to your sex arsenal; since it can keep going after you have come, you can always use it to finish off the work you've started. Or sometimes it can help with foreplay, getting your lover electrified and revved up before you get inside her. Toss it aside and end the play with your partner, at least for the first few times. This will remind both of you that the vibrator is just a fun novelty and not an essential.

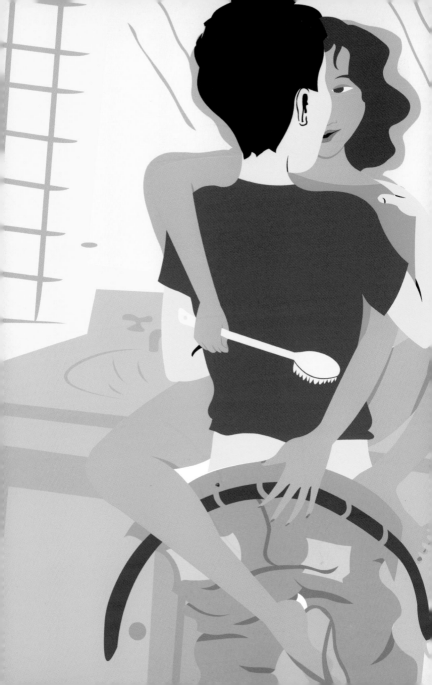

15 Minutes

In the time it takes to have a shower or even water the plants, you can treat your partner to a reminder of that electrical charge that first got you together. Try these scenarios to continue that important project you started long ago: to put the blush in the cheeks of your loved one.

Coffee-break Cunnilingus

If you're like most women, it takes about eight minutes to climax. Which means you should be able to accommodate two of life's pleasures—coffee and cunnilingus in a 15-minute break, mid-morning or mid-afternoon. So, take control of your man, but in a nice way: "I love it when . . ." rather than "I don't like that."

A few tips: Ask him to kiss from your stomach to your thighs, from your labia to your perineum (everywhere but your clit). He should start licking slowly and gently—teasingly, tauntingly soft and gentle. Tell him no matter how much you push and grind, he's to keep it light for the first few minutes before building up the pressure. He should also vary the strokes. Ask him to tongue each letter of the alphabet over your clit.

While you're heating up, your coffee should be cooling down. It is probably best not to indulge in both at the same time. Clutching a scalding cup of coffee while you are in paroxysms of pleasure will result in the wrong type of scream.

Slap and Tickle

Man, woman. Night, day. A kiss, a spank. Not only do opposites attract, they are also desirable. How does spanking cause sexual pleasure? It's all in the endorphin rush.

So when there is limited time to immerse yourself in pleasure, oddly enough, pain can get you there faster. But always begin with a tickle. Feathers are ideal, but anything soft and light can tickle—the petals of a flower, a silk scarf, a toothbrush, a soft hairbrush. Tease, torment, and tickle for five minutes. Swap the feather for a hand and give each butt cheek light slaps, slowly building the pressure. The rhythmic slapping should last for about five minutes, which leaves you five minutes more to get down to it.

Now, what did you say you were making for dinner?

Frantic Tantric

A Tantric quickie might seem like a contradiction, but even Sting will agree that a quickie can sexualize your whole day, stoking your inner fires and innate energy.

The technique of "kneeling at the gate of pleasure" works well if your lover's not initially hard, saving valuable wrist-work time. For this, you simply kneel and fondle him while he stands. After this good work is done, he should be on top and penetrate you before he is firmly erect.

Once inside you, he should lift your legs onto his shoulders and shift into a kneeling position. With your legs essentially supported by your shoulders, his hands are free. If you both like the sensation, he should insert one or two fingers inside you to massage your G-spot. His fingers not only stimulate the "sacred spot," but also his penis. A pleasant two-for-one time-saver, and the beginning of yoga time together.

Famous Blue Raincoat

Sometimes you can turn the element of surprise into instant foreplay. When you are picking up your lover for a night on the town or even, say, "date night," arrive wearing only a trench coat.

Don't hint that anything might be different. If you act natural, there might be no clue that you're naked underneath. Bring chilled champagne and say that before you go out, you want to celebrate some special occasion with a toast—it doesn't have to be anything big. Before the drink is served, open up your coat to reveal your sexy bod . . . and surprise! Stay there or move the glasses to the bedroom.

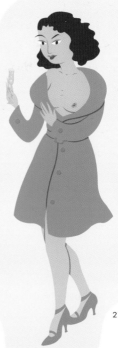

Voila! Instant seduction by surprise. It's a Hollywood classic because it works!

Chairs are hot. Along with the fireman's pole, they are strip-club standards. For his excitement, begin with one upright chair without arms. Make him sit and blindfold him, if you both like. Remove your clothes and use them (scarves, panties, stockings) to tie him to the chair. Straddle your man and rub against him, kissing him, slipping your nipples into his mouth. Get on your knees and be brilliantly succulent with his cock.

And if you have a swivel chair, this time the pleasure is yours. He's on his knees. Remove your panties, spread your legs, and ask him to softly swing the chair from side to side while his tongue seesaws your clit.

Yummy.

Rise and Shine

If you are both always on the go and your schedules are out of synch, you need to make the most of the morning. Sex first thing is fabulous because this is when our daily flow of hormones peak, hence your man's morning erection. Our bodies are also more relaxed after sleep and, as a result, more receptive.

So set his alarm 15 minutes before his usual wake-up. Don't tell him what you've done—a surreptitious, surprise shag will make his day. In fact, the first he should know of your plan is when he awakes to find his cock happily hardening in your mouth. In fact, there's no nicer way for you to be woken, too, so make sure he agrees to set your alarm another day.

Quietly then, mount your partner and ride him until the snooze button intervenes. As far as anyone else in the house is concerned, you're both still fast asleep. You'll both sport a warm glow for the rest of the day.

Take it to the Floor

When an opportunity for a quickie presents itself, grab it, no matter how uncomfortable it may appear. Cement floors aren't really that bad once you focus on the fun you're about to have. And while bruised knees are not attractive, they carry a certain erotic cachet.

To do it right without causing scars, bruises, or any accompanying pain, you both need to kneel on something. In the absence of a yoga mat or cushions, slip off your shoes and wedge your knees into them. Ask him to knead your ass and play with your pussy, to get you warm-red and ready for rear entry. He should play with your breasts and you his balls.

Once he's deep inside you, bring your legs together and squeeze slowly and gently. This way you get more stimulation, he gets tighter thrusts, and he'll promise to be yours forever.

Heavenly Petting

When we're insanely busy, it's easy to skip first, second, and even third base, and just aim for home runs. But have you forgotten the exquisite fun of necking in the park, groping at parties and fondling each other on the sofa? Put penetration on the backburner and spend 15 minutes getting back to basics.

Your hormones may not be partying as energetically this time around, but your technique has really improved! The breast/nipple orgasm is common for women. Ask him to circle the skin around your nipple, gradually closing in until just his index finger and thumb are spiraling your erect nipples. Then he should follow the same motion with his tongue.

Find out if his nipples are directly linked to his dick. As you get hot, use ice cubes on each other to cool down, elicit shivers, and to stiffen nipples. Face each other, kneeling on the floor, and indulge in some mutual pleasuring.

Suck it and See

This super-deluxe blow-job technique should last the full 15 minutes—just enough time to make it famous in his erotic memory.

Tease him first by kissing everywhere but where he's desperate for you to go. Then hold the base of his cock and in the lightest, gentlest way. Take the head, just the head, into your mouth and, keeping the tip of your tongue soft, tenderly lick the tip. Tease him like this for a while.

Once the head is well-lubricated, gently slip your thumb and forefinger around the head, moving up and down slowly while you continue to lick the tip. As you begin to slide your mouth further down his shaft, imagine your mouth is a hot, tight, wet pussy. Keep it firm around him and let it enter slowly, even with some effort, as if your mouth were a virgin!

Start to pump his penis rhythmically with your hand and mouth, using your other hand to stroke his perineum. Wet your finger and edge towards his anus before circling his hole and slowly slipping your finger into him. His G-spot, roughly 3 inches inside him, is the quickest route to his heart.

Party Animals

The party's swinging, and the hosts are delighted to see you both. After a few drinks, you think how lucky you are to have such a fabulous lover. If it's your first visit, ask the host for a tour, so you can scope out a location. If you need an excuse, say you're getting more drinks.

Never use the bathroom—someone will come knocking. Instead, try up against the door of a bedroom to prevent intrusion. Or scout outside for a dark, isolated corner.

Before he enters you, spend some time rubbing his cock between your pussy lips. If there's no lube at hand, make sure you use plenty of saliva so it's nice and slippery.

Once you've finished, don't forget to reappear with whatever you said you were going to fetch—the highballs or cocktails!

Bend Overtime

There is something deliciously decadent about violating the sanctified space of his workplace. So take action and slip into stockings and a skirt, pack a vibrator in your handbag, and head full speed to his office at a time when everyone else is going home. Let him know you're coming with some nourishment and you won't stay longer than 15 minutes.

Sit on his desk, telling him to stay seated in his chair in front of you. Slowly part your legs so that he glimpses your stockings, then reach for your vibrator. Tell him you'd like to give him an hors d'oeuvre before his main course, which is waiting for him at home.

Slide back so your pussy is at the edge of the desk and ask him to lick your clit while slowly pushing the vibrator deeper and deeper inside you. Once you've come—and the tongue/vibrator is so delicious it shouldn't take long—flip over and stick your bottom in the air. Gyrate in a come-nether fashion. Let him have a few thrusts inside you—but only a few. Then withdraw, pack up your things, and expect him home early.

Aural Sex

Never underestimate the power of your phone. Talk dirty to keep things hot between you and your lover. Tell him in very specific terms exactly what you would like to do to him and have him do to you. Describe your body; and your virtues. It sounds cliché, but describe what you're wearing and be sure to be wearing something extra sexy. Give your man something he can picture in his mind and then transfer to his glans!

Don't race. Slow it down and listen for the heavy breathing. A pause lets the other person fill in the picture.

One famous technique is the erotic cliffhanger. Call when you know he or she can't answer, and go into graphic detail about what you'd like to do to them right now or tomorrow or next week, and then expect to be cut off by the machine or voicemail. That way, you'll be the priority call back when the message is picked up.

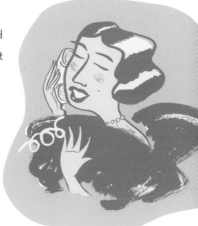

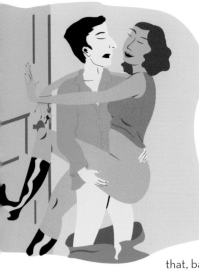

You were dripping with desire during your evening out. Yet somehow, once you got home, let the dog out, checked in on a sleeping child or three, and took off your makeup, the moment had passed.

Avoid domestic distractions by making a commitment to your partner that, barring the presence of the babysitter, you'll screw the second you get through the door.

While still traveling home, describe what you will do to him when you get him indoors. Encourage him to speak up also. This way you will know exactly what your partner wants that night, curtailing possible frustration. To exploit the mental foreplay, make sure you engage in a full-bodied, fabulous French kiss before you follow through with your just-planned activities.

Backseat Driver

Instead of leaving for an evening out five minutes late, try setting off 15 minutes early. Depending on your urge to outrage public decency and end up behind bars, pull into a relatively secluded spot. While en route, if he is driving, you should remove your knickers, place your legs on the dashboard and start masturbating. You should also provide a running commentary to your partner as you engage your clit and pussy with your fingers, which should prompt him to switch off the sports scores on the radio.

Once you park, he should scramble first onto the back seat. Facing away from him, sit on his lap with your knees either side of his thighs and clutch the seats in front of you while you bounce up and down. This position lets you to control the depth and speed of the thrusts as well as the overall timing. And you get to be a backseat driver without the complaining.

Freshly Squeezed Juices

He's too busy to eat breakfast, so surprise him with breakfast in bed!

Get an orange (or any other soft fruit) and cut off one end just smaller than his cock. Note: This works best at room temperature! You can cut a hole all the way through to the other side, leaving just the skin on. Squeeze it around his cock and start jerking him off. If he's more of a mango man, cut a ripe mango in half, remove the seed and eat the soft flesh with a spoon. Leave a thin layer of mango flesh on the skins. Use this to masturbate him. The sensation is fantastic and the bonus is that his cock will taste nice and fruity!

Try other variations, such a cucumbers. Clean the middle out of it, place his cock in it, and twist in a clockwise motion. Things may get messy, so you'll want to lay down a towel beforehand to soak up any spilled juices. What a fabulous way to start the day.

Close Shave

Busy couples combine grooming and foreplay into a single act because nothing beats the electric frisson of smooth skin on smooth skin. Another advantage to trimmed pubes is there that there is less hair to get in the way during oral sex.

Use an electric trimmer or shaver, which has several advantages over a razor blade—the main one being it won't nick or cut. There are no razor burn or bumps. And of course, there are the vibrations!

Men will always get a hard-on when having their pubes shaved, even if you make sure not to touch his cock. If you actually touch his cock with the vibrating shaver, it won't be long before he erupts. As for women, running the warm, vibrating shaver over her pussy should really get her juices flowing. Because you won't need lather or water, you can shave anywhere—including bed—without making much of a mess!

Ice-cream Oral

Make oral sex better for you and for him with some ice-cream. But don't just spoon it on—buy an ice-cream cone, bite off the end and slip it over his still-soft penis. Now add the ice-cream and take your time nibbling and licking until he's so hard that he breaks out of the cone! Or, pop a popsicle or frozen berries in your mouth instead.

Men can prod and poke into new territory around their partner's pussy lips and clit with their frozen tongue tips. The surprise sensation will shock and arouse your partner to new heights. And their own sexy taste will be enhanced with Ben and Jerry's!

After you've tried this technique a few times, try filling your mouth with warm tea or hot chocolate immediately afterwards. They won't know what hit them when the temperature goes from arctic to tropical. Either way, this should get you both screaming in no time.

Black Rain

Save time on morning showers by taking a sexy evening shower together in the dark. Being in the dark will heighten your sense of touch. Once you have her in the shower, wash her body gently and sensually. Begin scrubbing her from behind and work your way down to her butt, the back of her thighs, her calves, and even her feet. And while you're kneeling down, turn her around and begin working your way up from her shins to her stomach and finally, her breasts. Don't neglect her arms, her neck and of course, put some soap on your hand to adequately clean her pussy.

If you think you have the stamina or strength, hold her up against the tiles, let her wrap her legs around your waist and start to grind inside her. Let the water splash against your bodies while you're making love.

If you'd like to watch her get crazy wet and wild, lie in the tub and let her ride you like a trouper. What could possibly be better?

Stand and Deliver

Doing a spot of spring cleaning? Sick of the boredom of household chores? Any time you are both vertical is the perfect time for stand-up sex. Drop that vacuum cleaner and get to it!

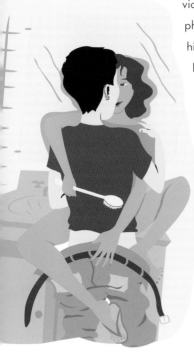

If your guy's got a few inches on you (or vice versa), stand on a step or a phone book. Have your man bend his knees to lower himself a bit so he can enter you and then rise up. For yogis and athletes, stand on one leg and hook the other around him. You may not have a great range of motion, but he can make waves by rocking you back and forth. You can also lean against a wall, put your arms around his neck, have him lift you by holding onto your thighs or locking his hands beneath your butt, and wrap your legs around his hips.

Hit and Missionary

You know you're fighting over something petty that isn't getting resolved. Sometimes the best way to make up quickly is to stop talking and ask him to get on top of you and make "body love." We want to feel like we're at the center of our partners' world, and what better way to show each other just that than to make love to the whole of their body with the whole of yours? This is why the missionary is such a classic.

Your man should not rest his full weight on top of you, but support himself with his forearms, as if doing push-ups. One drawback to this position is the lack of direct stimulation to your clit. If you need more, ask him to press in closer to you and grind your clit against his pelvis. He should move slowly and use short, deep thrusts. Take advantage of the romance and intimacy this position allows by whispering sweet nothings in your partner's ear or nibbling a tongue or earlobe.

If you're still not getting enough stimulation, put your legs up over his shoulders so his cock will connect with your G-Spot. Keep using your hands to touch, caress, and explore. The missionary is so powerful at reviving intimacy that afterwards you'll have forgotten why you were arguing in the first place.

Massage the Figures

Sometimes one of you is in the right mood but the other isn't. What's a fast way to get your partner aroused? Offer a quick massage, to de-stress. Put your partner's favorite music on (within reason—no Sex Pistols or Guns N' Roses) to help them relax into a mellow state. Pour a generous amount of massage oil into your palm and rub your hands together lightly. When both hands are warm, apply long, deep strokes to your partner's back, chest, arms, and hands. Once your partner is relaxed, you can start the sexy part of the massage!

Guys should start by gently rubbing her entire vulva, followed with clitoral stimulation, and finishing with internal and clitoral stimulation. Stimulate the G-Spot with first and then second fingers together. He should then close his fingers rhythmically inside your pussy (signaling to "come here").

Massaging your man's nether region is about slowing down and stopping, or changing your actions, just before the point of no return. Vary your strokes at first, and then concentrate on one or two kinds of strokes as you come close to the end. By bringing your lover to the peak without allowing release, you prolong his hard-on, resulting in a more intense orgasm.

Knotty Delight

Quickie sex means always upping your game sexually. After discussing some of your partner's fantasies, you might want to explore a very common one—some type of light bondage.

If you're comfortable with your partner and total trust has been established, just ask her or him if they want to be tied up lightly. (You definitely don't want to surprise them with this one.) With their permission, you can first try tying their hands together. Something as simple as a light kiss on the cheek is different with someone's hands tied together loosely!

Next you can try adding their feet, further restricting their movement. Being more helpless can add greatly to their erotic excitement and experience. Always be careful not to tie your partner too tightly, however. You want to get the blood pumping rather than impair circulation.

Undress to Impress

First, choose the song—something you love, and one you know you can move to. If you're dancing for your woman, how about a song that means something to both of you? Next, focus on the final layer—the one you will reveal last. Now is the time to pick up one of those sexy boy-thongs to surprise her.

Now sit your woman down and turn out the lights, leaving just few candles to light up the show. Start your music and strut out there. Sway, and start to undo your outer layer. Show your sweetie your to-die-for backside. Tease. Flash her, then quickly close your shirt. Spin around and show her some tantalizing angles. Get close to her—so close she can smell you—but she can't touch yet. Remember to toss her your garments.

Once you're down to your final layer, go even slower: Lower your boxers, briefs, or G-string almost all the way down before pulling them back up. Put your hands behind your head. Flex your biceps to cover up your belly (or flaunt your sixpack). Put your hands on your knees and wiggle your butt in a wave-like motion. Dance seductively, tantalizingly, and roll each sock down your leg. Slide your shoes off and, if you've done a good job, she'll have her own clothes off in a fraction of the time it took you!

Let's Get Hitched

For those of you already wed, here's an opportunity to renew your vows. Or, if you have yet to tie the knot, consider this a fun game where you can have a trial run.

Any wedding takes a bit of planning so here's what you need:

> 1 cock ring (available at any reputable sex or condom store)
>
> 1 bottle champagne (no vows are complete without a celebratory toast)

After a quick toast, undress each other completely. Whether he is hard or not, you can each ask the crucial question of the other and let one of you be responsible for slipping the ring on his cock.

With the ceremony over, there's still the cake, of course. Or you could skip straight to whipped cream all over your lover's genitals. Tasty. You can now consummate, and voila—an entire wedding ceremony in mere minutes instead of months. This is one ceremony where you should keep your garter on for maximum effect!

Hotel Californication

This is a decadent quickie for the occupationally mismatched couple—a lunchtime liaison in a hotel room. Find a hotel close to your work or his and ask for a short-stay rate. After all, you'll be in and out in less than half an hour. On a day when you're sure neither of you will be needed in the boardroom, tell your partner that you need them for a quick lunch break. Say it's urgent and has to be in person.

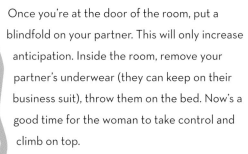

Once you're at the door of the room, put a blindfold on your partner. This will only increase anticipation. Inside the room, remove your partner's underwear (they can keep on their business suit), throw them on the bed. Now's a good time for the woman to take control and climb on top.

Once you get down to sex, the woman should rest her hands behind her on the man's thighs and arch her back. Then she can slide up and down him, with her ass ass supported by his hands—this position really hits the G-Spot. Then a quick freshen up and you're both back to work.

Naked Canvas

Busy couples can be artists and lovers at the same time with body paint. So if your partner is up for it, why not satisfy your urge to paint a Picasso in less time then it takes a real artist to choose paints?

Body paints come in all kinds of colors and delicious flavors, so you can paint your lover's body and then lick it off ravenously. Use brushes, sponges, or even your fingers to create different impressions. Paint something that teases your partner with varied brush strokes around various parts of their body. It's tempting, but be sure not to attack their erogenous zones straight away. Let your creativity sparkle! You can heighten your lover's sense of touch by blindfolding them. This way they won't know what's coming when, and you'll turn a feat of the visual arts into the peak of the sensual arts.

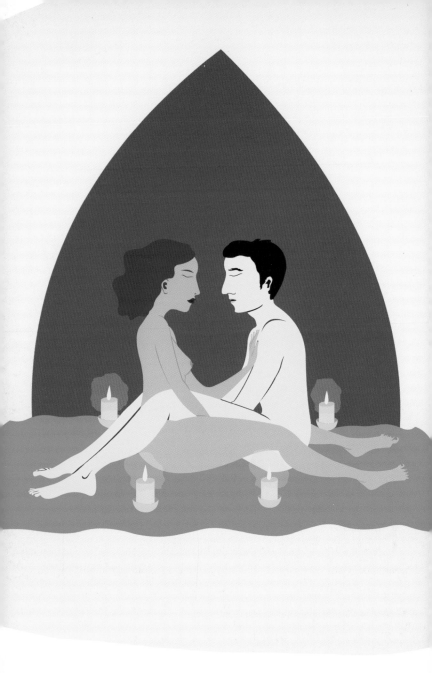

30 Minutes

The motto of the adventurous, successful, and multiorgasmic has long been "carpe diem." So seize that next half-hour you have alone with your lover. Instead of merely discussing the best and worst of your day so far, imagine the evening ahead after you've followed one of these scenarios. You'll be gazing through the gorgeous rose-tinted glasses that only a great orgasm can give.

Assume the Position (or Three)

Fight off those "God, this is the same old, same old" thoughts by going wild with three different positions in one session. Half an hour gives you plenty of time to have sex three ways—just warn your man he's in for a serious workout.

Start in an "old faithful" position you know and love, but after 10 minutes, flip each other into a new position. And after another 10 minutes, it's all change again. The following combinations work well and shouldn't be too much hard work for either of you. Let's get physical!

Doggy Style to Flat Doggy to Spooning: Start on all fours with your bloke kneeling behind you, thrusting. Move to Flat Doggy by collapsing onto the bed, so that you're both lying flat, with him on top of you. For extra stimulation, slip your hand between your legs and rub your clit, or cup his balls. Finally, both of you roll together so that you're lying on your sides, gently rocking your way to orgasm.

Missionary to the Neck Lock to the Shoulder Stand: Start with him on top then, after 10 minutes, raise your legs up to wrap them around his neck. If he lifts your legs and supports them this is way easier. Finally, slide your hands under your hips to raise them up, leaning back so that you're supporting your entire body weight on your shoulders. This gets seriously deep penetration (so it's particularly good if he's not that well endowed).

Cowgirl to Reverse CAT to Facing Spoons: Start on top of your bloke, facing him. After riding him for 10 minutes, flop forwards to lie flat on top of him, wriggling down so that your clit is rubbing against his pubic bone, with him still inside you. And for your last move, simply roll together so you're facing each other and finish the job!

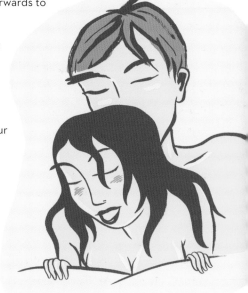

Candid Camera

Grab your digital camera or video camera for a seriously hot foreplay session that can start before your other half gets home. By the time you've made a sexy video, and he's watched it, both of you will be desperate to rip off your clothes and get down to it. Even better, the vid can double up as a reminder of you when you're apart—you can guarantee he'll use it. And let's face it, someone masturbating about you is one of the best compliments ever.

A bit of practical consideration makes all the difference. Put the camera on a tripod so that it doesn't wobble. If you're using a camera phone, judicious use of adhesive tape to prop it up can help. Put on your sexiest outfit—a slinky dress with your sexiest underwear underneath (when he returns the favor, it's a good excuse to get him into—and out of—a tux).

Start your on-screen seduction with a sexy striptease. Run your hands all over your body, looking at each body part as you touch it, then look straight into camera. Once you're naked—or wearing just a few carefully selected pieces of underwear—start to masturbate. As well as being hot to watch, it will show your man how you really like to be touched. You can end with an orgasm, or save that for him to deliver . . .

Once your video is made, deliver it to your lover with a message attached reading: "This is just the beginning . . ." Then wait for him to turn up on your doorstep desperate for more.

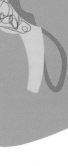

Come Again

Like the idea of having an orgasm so intense it leaves you shaking? Well, why have one orgasm when you can have two? Take it in turns to do this to each other—it'll be two 30-minute sessions well spent.

Men: Give her a clitoral orgasm followed by a G-Spot orgasm. Oral sex is the easiest way to make her come through her clit. Women usually prefer much lighter pressure to men, so lick as gently as you possibly can, tracing your tongue over the labia and thighs as well as the clit.

Once she's come, stop touching her clit—it'll be much too sensitive. Slide one or two fingers deep inside her and feel for her G-spot (on the upper wall of the vagina about 3 or 4 inches in). You'll feel this start to swell. Press very firmly upwards and rock your hand. With any luck, it will swell more—press harder as it does and you should be able to make her come and ejaculate all at once.

Women: Throw out your squeamishness and go for a prostate orgasm, then the old-fashioned version. Start by covering your finger in lubricant, then circle the anus softly. Warn your man first—otherwise he'll clench up, which is the last thing you need. As he relaxes, rest your finger firmly against the rim, then increase the pressure and you should find his anus opening up for you. Slip your finger in slowly until you feel the prostate (a walnut-shaped lump 2 or 3 inches inside the anus), then press firmly against it. As you stroke you should feel it (and him) start to swell. He'll start to tingle and get intense feelings running through his body. He may ejaculate but that's not necessary for him to have an orgasm, and with any luck, he won't as that makes it easier for you to make him come using traditional methods afterwards. Go for a blow job or (after washing your hands) a hand job to take him over the edge.

He won't be able to wipe the smile off his face for weeks!

Rewards and Punishment

Think tying someone up is the kinkiest way to do bondage? Think again. Tonight you're going to dominate your man without digging out any props. You can guarantee that it's much more intense restricting your man's movements using his mind alone. And hell, you get to be bossy, which is no bad thing.

Order your man to lie on the bed and say you're going to position him as you want him. (You may need to reassure him that you won't stand him up in front of a pile of dirty dishes). Once he's in position, he's not allowed to move, no matter what you do. You can add a threat—say, of a spanking—if he doesn't do exactly as he's told. Then spread his legs and pin his arms over his head.

Now start to tease him mercilessly. Kneel across his body, facing his feet. Starting at his feet, kiss them all over. Run your tongue over his toes and instep. If he's got ticklish feet, massage his feet with firm pressure first to desensitize them a little. Work your way up the ankles (the outside of the ankle about 2 inches up from the foot is a sexy acupressure point), the legs, inner thighs, and cock. But only pause briefly there before moving up the stomach, chest, nipples, neck, ears, and lips. By now, he'll probably be desperate to press against you, so reinforce his inability to move by pinning his arms above his head as you kiss him.

Then work back down—slowly—to his genitals and finish with a steamy oral sex session. Or, if you're feeling really mean, masturbate over his face, giving them a close-up view of a very personal act. Tell him that if he's really good, you'll make him come afterwards, but he has to stay absolutely still and keep his hands to himself.

Expect serious orgasms from this one—the best sex really is all in the mind.

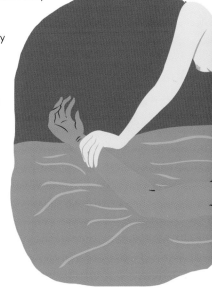

Synchronicity

Go for a sensual Eastern session—silk drapes and lute player optional—by having a Tantric taster session. If you initiate it with your partner, she'll think you're the most sensual lover in the world, which has got to be worth some brownie points. And the good news is that Tantra isn't always about seven-hour marathons. It's entirely possible to have a sensual Tantric experience in 30 minutes. The important thing to bear in mind is that Tantra is more about connection than sex—though the orgasms are utterly intense if you build a strong enough connection.

Start by putting on some relaxing music, lighting some candles, and shedding your clothes. Now, sit facing your partner and look into her eyes. You may get an urge to laugh. If so, go with it— just relax and enjoy the intimacy. After five minutes, move closer, part your lips, and start inhaling your partner's breath and letting her breathe yours. Synchronizing your breathing will build intensity (though stop if either of you become dizzy).

After five minutes of breathing together, touch your palms to each other's and, still gazing into one another's eyes, feel the warmth of your partner's skin and the flow of energy between you. Do this for five minutes then move on to a chakra massage.

There are seven chakras. Your root chakra is between your anus and genitals (your perineum). Next comes the orange chakra in the center of your abdomen. Moving up, you then have the solar plexus, heart, and throat chakras, which are self-explanatory. After that comes your brow chakra/third eye, between your eyes in the center of your forehead, and finally your crown chakra, which is on the top of your head in the center of your scalp.

To give a chakra massage, run your fingers from one chakra to the next, working from the root to the crown. Allow 10 minutes each for this, though you could spend a lot longer if you had more time. By the time you finish, you'll both be utterly connected and so turned on that the remaining five minutes will entail super-charged sex.

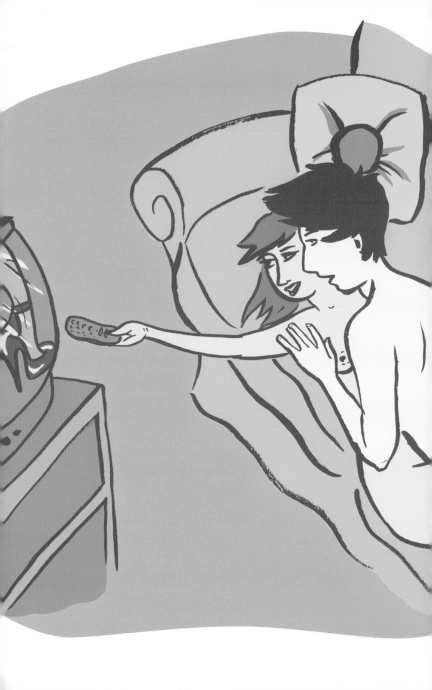

Sure-fire Shortcuts

We love shortcuts because it encourages our competitive spirits—not only do we love the idea of getting somewhere faster, we love the idea that the knowledge is our little secret! These shortcuts take the value of your time into account fully, so when you finally get together for a quickie, you'll both be secretly full of anticipation—and as hot and wet as the summer rain outside.

Raise the Stakes

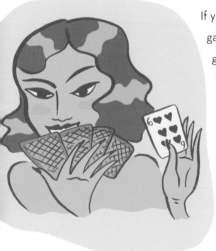

If you love cards or board games, this little shortcut will get you out of the game and into the bedroom faster than you can say "roll again!"

Sexy Scrabble: Play using only sensual and erotic words. You may need to loosen the rules slightly and use more than seven letters at a time.

Rename the countries in Risk as body parts on the board, so when you take over a "body part" you get to have your way with it for five minutes.

Chess: Every time you take over a partner's piece you are entitled to five minutes of a romantic "treat" of your choice.

Or take a deck of cards. Assign each card a thing to do. For example, kings are a long, hot kiss; aces mean oral sex; and the Joker is "anything goes"! Shuffle the deck, spread out the cards, and take turns to draw.

In a Pinch

One way to make your partner come faster is by stepping up the intensity of your touching during your lovemaking. Try light scratching, biting, or pinching. Not enough to hurt, of course, but enough to wake up your lover's senses. In each case, start very lightly and intensify the pressure gradually. If you think of a range of 1 to 10, with 1 signifying a touch that you can barely feel and 10 being painful, stay in the 1-5 range. The gentle bite or pinching of nipples for men and women usually produces a warm sensation in our sex organs and gets our juices flowing. A key part of this shortcut is the surprise factor, so it is important not to go overboard with the sensation—this is not about hurting your partner. If you feel yourself on the verge of coming and feel your partner might be lagging behind, double up on the intensity, pinch, scratch, or bite that much harder—and help to trigger your partner's orgasm.

More-gasmic

The day of your next hot date, run off to the Ladies when you get the chance and masturbate. Not so that you come, just enough to get you lubricated. Do this as often as possible. Why? Because every time you do, you'll be sending blood down towards your pussy, revving up your nerve endings and making you much more likely to have a multiple orgasm when you eventually have sex. You'll be "More-gasmic." Use the first two fingers of your right hand, with your clit nestled between them. Move the fingers in a round-and-round motion. Repeat all day. But warn your date: You're going to be almost illegally aroused by the time you meet.

Knickerbocker Glorious

What panties should you wear for instant passion? Ones that tie on the sides. Do them up with a gentle bow and they'll fall off with a flick of his wrist. Otherwise, opt for flimsy G-strings and thongs, which are not only more arousing but he can nudge them to one side should the need arise. And of course, French panties, *ouvert*, with the built-in slit designed for easy access, are ideal for *les liaisons dangereuses*. If you wear panties as well as stockings and suspenders, you can whip them off in a striptease and still keep the sexy fishnets on as he ravishes you. Or wear just a slip instead. A good half-slip will never come between you and your man. When you're out, tell him you forgot your panties and invite him to touch you. If you're doing everything right, he won't need an invitation to the after-party.

Raise Your Game

When you need to condense an hour worth of passion into a five- or 15-minute slot, you don't have time to simmer gently before reaching a boil. Ideally, you'd go from cold to hot in less time than it takes to make a cup of tea. It's easier for men, of course. They are ready for action before the kettle has even boiled. But by upping the ante physically, you will stimulate your senses more readily. Show your need and give into the passion. Be firm. Swap caresses for scratches. Grab instead of rub. Spank rather than massage. Bite instead of kiss. So if you'd normally nibble each other's neck or lips, start using your teeth and give little bites. Instead of licking nipples, introduce a hint of teeth and some gentle biting to quickly bring them to attention. The philosophy? Get out of your mind and into your senses by engaging them without fear, quickly and intensely.

5ex Me55aging

Anticipating pleasure is a form of pleasure itself. Being drip-fed sexy text messages intermittently throughout the day is a major tease. It's also easy foreplay with barely lifting a finger. The messages should be unexpected and dirty enough to cause a sharp intake of breath and a shooting surge of excrutiating passion from heart to hardening desire and back again. Use your intimate knowledge of your partner's fantasies to ensure the messages hit their target. If you have total faith in your partner's discretion, you could send him a few picture messages, each one revealing a little more than the one before. Tormenting texts and images only take a few seconds to send, but their cumulative effect should increase anticipation throughout the day, so you can end your day with a bang!

Try these text-message shortcuts:

brb—be right back	f2p—free to play
bg—big grin	lol—laugh out loud
cm—call me	l8r—later
njoy—enjoy	pc—pussy

Inter-lube

You wouldn't make an egg salad sandwich without mayonnaise.
Greens without dressing are downright dull. How would your
car function without oil? Lube always makes things better and
sex is no exception. For women, one drawback of quickies is in-
sufficient time to lubricate naturally. We don't always have time
to be slowly and sensuously aroused until we're dripping, yet
the rules for good sex are non-negotiable: He's got to be hard
and you've got to be wet. A drop of lube is often the answer.
Generally speaking, a woman can never be too wet, so keep
some lube under your bed and in your handbag at all times.
There are lots of silky lubricants on the market, including hot
fudge sundae, strawberry- or banana-flavored water-soluble
lubricant, just in case your sweetie needs further sweetening.

Day Stripper

So what clothes facilitate "anytime, anyplace" action when you're in a rush? A tight pair of jeans might look sexy but they're about as conducive for a quickie as your period. Skirts and dresses are far more lust-friendly. We look more feminine, feel sexier, and they lend themselves perfectly—both practically and visually—to impromptu orgasms. Although garter belts are also ideal for fast action, what busy woman has time in the morning to fish around for a suspender belt, fiddle with fasteners, and find a pair of matching stockings? Why not buy 10 identical pairs of thigh-high stockings that hold themselves up, in order to obtain the look without the hassle? Want a new jacket? Think again—a long raincoat is more practical. To any passer-by you look like you're hugging and kissing. In fact, your skirt is up around your waist while he is lodged firmly inside you.

Good Vibrations

A vibrator is the quickest way to go from "Oh no, no" to "Oh God, yes, yes, YES!" But you have to learn where to apply it. Don't simply clamp it over your clit and expect instant gratification. Your clit is delicate and if you batter it about, you'll only deaden the nerves and add hours to starting your arousal. Instead, try the off-center pleasure move: Turn your vibrator to its lowest speed and move it around the very outside edge of your clit. After a minute, move it inwards until it's touching one side of the clitoris. Mmm . . . feels good, doesn't it? Now turn the speed up a notch and work it so its tip is rubbing up and down the edge of your clit. As soon as you feel you're about to explode, touch your clit directly, full-force, with your vibrator on top speed. Bam! You've come and the batteries in your vibrator are still fully charged.

Stiff Competition

Penises are temperamental. One minute they're drilling a hole through your back with urgency, the next they're as limp as a wet noodle. Since we can't always secrete on demand, we must forgive men when they can't summon an erection. If you want it and want it now, you need to do something. To get him standing awake and erect, when all it wants to do is lounge and nestle, fierce tugging won't help. Instead, tease him by lightly stroking his cock, brushing his balls, and tickling his upper thighs. Trail your fingertips over his cock every now and then until you feel it twitching with need. Another foolproof method of getting wood involves a generous squeeze of lubrication. It transforms a common or garden-variety hand job into such a mind-blowing, super-deluxe version that when, at a later date, you offer "hand or mouth," some wavering will absolutely follow.

Hanky Spanky

There is an art to spanking. Spanking is a life skill, like being able to change a tire or make chicken soup, and it is bound to come in useful. For starters, you can always use it on a partner when one of you is too tired to perform but doesn't mind exercising the odd arm muscle. The easiest way to administer spanks is with a paddle (a wooden instrument like a table tennis bat). If you are spanking, you should take control and bend him over, pulling down his boxers. You should stand closely behind so he can feel you against your bottom. You should run your hands up his back and body. You should connect with him, make him feel safe—trust is crucial. Intimacy should flow from your fingertips into him. You should build up strokes gently, achieving a steady rhythm. If using your hand, cup instead of use the flat of your palm, and alternate between teasing and tormenting. The sacral crease, where the buttocks meet the thigh (known as "the sweet spot"), is the most sensuous. Sometimes you really have to be cruel to be kind.

Shower Head

If you've never used a shower head for impure motives, now's your chance. Two types of shower head are preferable for good, clean, dirty fun. One is where you can unscrew the diffuser top so that a jet shoots out rather than a sprinkle. The other is a shower head with massage settings, including a vibrating option.

Find a comfortable position and make sure the temperature of the water is warm rather than hot. Start with low pressure and very gradually step up it up. Try directing the water onto different points—you may find a direct stream onto your clit intensely erotic, or you may prefer a flutter of water over your labia (but don't spray it up the vagina as this can be dangerous). Try squatting and letting the jet shoot onto your clit from above—a sensation akin to being licked by a man with a vibrating tongue. However, don't focus all the attention between your legs, as the sensual spray hitting other parts of your body is deliciously stimulating too.

CAT-Woman

Nothing quite matches the contentment of both of you grinning like Cheshire cats at the close of proceedings. The Coital Alignment Technique, or CAT position, increases the chance of female orgasms through intercourse from 23 to 77 percent, as well as upping the odds of simultaneous orgasm. To try it, ask your man to rest his full weight on you and then edge forward so his pelvis is directly over yours. Wrap your legs around his thighs, rest your ankles on his calves and rock gently against each other's pelvis. Push upward and forward so that your clit makes contact with the base of his cock. Establish a gentle and natural rhythm. As orgasm approaches, don't speed up, just keep gently rocking. Your orgasm will arrive naturally. You and the cat who got the cream should end up with a great deal in common.

The Venus Butterfly

If you want a shortcut to get her to come, go straight to the source—the clitoris. The clit has thousands upon thousands of nerve endings. Like your cock, when she is aroused, it becomes more rigid as it fills with blood. You will want to respect that her clit is her most sensitive body part. Rough rubbing or licking directly on it (especially with rough skin or too much vigor) is rarely the ideal. She will want constant, repetitive motion to one or both sides of her clit. Women usually have a favorite side, so it is always good to ask which side your baby likes. Expose her clit by spreading her lips and lightly pulling back her hood. With her clit exposed, give it a quick little suck. Do not use your teeth or use heavy suction when starting out. Suck outside the clit so your tongue bends in a V. Go slow. Try gently nibbling her labia. Pull on them lightly, until she makes a sound. Then lick and suck around her clit but not the clit itself. Wait until she begs. Note that pulling back the hood is very personal. The more a woman is aroused, the more she may want or not want her clitoris stimulated directly. Make sure you discuss this beforehand. As well, remember that after an orgasm the clit can retract, and becomes highly sensitive to any further stimulation, often to the point of being painful.

Fast Foreplay

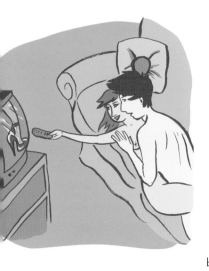

Let's admit it, watching porn makes you wet and him hard. So if you as so busy you want instant foreplay, just watching some porn or erotica together should act as a sure-fire shortcut!

There is a huge variety out there—soft-core, hard-core, porn that claims to be "artsy" or tasteful. Pick some up—really grab anything, it doesn't matter since the point is you'll only be watching it for a few minutes. It's on simply to get you aroused. Turn up the sound, because hearing someone else have fun increases our desire. The films usually contain around six sex scenes, appealing to the widest audience. You might see a couple, threesomes, two women, orgies, anal, oral, and various positions. If a particular scene isn't doing it for the two of you, hit "fast forward." Once you're both aching to get out of your clothes, strip and follow suit.

Squeeze Play

Some women can achieve sexual pleasure—even orgasm—by simply squeezing or rubbing their thighs together. No secret here—this indirectly stimulates their clitoris. You can use this discreet technique anywhere, even in public! Long train ride? Boring desk job? Now's your chance to have fun en route to or at work! Never tried it? You might want to practice at home by lying flat, locking your ankles together. Now rhythmically squeeze your thighs together, fantasize, and occasionally touch your nipples if you are having difficulty reaching orgasm by thigh-squeezing alone. Another technique is to cross your legs and tuck an ankle around the other leg, which creates pressure on the clitoral area. Some women seem to prefer "riding the seam" of jeans; others like the greater closeness of pantyhose or bare legs under a skirt or dress. Experiment and find what works best for you. Careful, though—if you get carried away and perfect this technique, you run the risk of being turned on any time you sit!

"Sex is not the answer.
Sex is the question.
Yes is the answer."

— Howard Hoffman

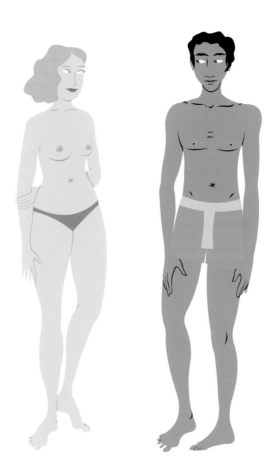